MENTAL HEALTH PRIMER

Thomas Moll BA RN,BC CPMHN(C) CCHP

Copyright © 2018 Thomas Moll

All rights reserved

ISBN: 1720510571

ISBN-13: 978-1720510574

Contents

Introduction to Psych 4
The DSM and the Multiaxial Diagnosis 5
The Psychiatric Consultation 8
The MSE 11
Schizophrenia 18
Hallucinations and Diagnosis 21
Antipsychotic Medication 23
Major Depressive Disorder 25
Antidepressants 26
Bipolar Disorder 30
Pharmacological Treatment for Bipolar Disorder 32
Benzodiazepines 34
Generalized Anxiety Disorder 36
Personality Disorders 37
Cluster A Personality Disorders "The Mad" 38
   The Paranoid PD 39
   The Schizoid PD 39
   The Schizotypal PD 40
Cluster B Personality Disorders "The Bad" 41
   The Antisocial PD 41

- The Borderline PD 43
- The Histrionic PD 44
- The Narcissistic PD 45

Cluster C Personality Disorders "The Sad" 46
- The Avoidant PD 46
- The Dependent PD 47
- The Obsessive-Compulsive PD 48
- The Depressive PD 49

Mental Health Providers 50

Treatment Modalities 51

Cross Cultural Psychiatry 53

Resources 56

Mental Health Terms 57

Introduction to Psych

Psychiatry and behavioral health can be a mysterious field, even to health professionals. Most physicians and nurses receive little education regarding mental health (MH) during their standard training and it can be a daunting task to work with and understand patients with mental illnesses. The purpose of this primer is to give a foundation of understanding of this field. We will first learn the basics of how to "talk the talk" of mental health and then delve into the most often encountered mental health diseases and conditions along with the different modalities of treatment including medications.

The first point of entry for many people to a mental health record is the psychiatric consultation. Often it is filled with psychiatric-specific terms and is either skipped over by the reader or just the final plan is read. As a young student nurse, in my psychiatric rotation, I asked my instructor questions regarding the diagnostic system used in the psych consult. I was told to skip reading the psych consult, "It's too complicated. That's just for psychiatrists. You don't need to know that stuff." It's not too complicated, everyone can understand it, and we all benefit from knowing more about a patient's mental health.

The fundamental starting point for psychiatrists is the **Mental Status Exam** (MSE). Similar to a Review of Systems (ROS) performed by our more medically oriented providers, the MSE is the clinical snapshot of the patient's current state of mind. The MSE is a standardized way of painting the psychiatric clinical picture, as we will see.

The DSM and the Multiaxial Diagnosis

The theoretical framework for mental health practice is the **Diagnostic and Statistical Manual (DSM)**. This massive tome was first published in 1952 and listed about 60 different disorders. It has been revised many times, every ten years or so. The current revision, DSM-5, was published in 2013 but many clinicians continue to use the DSM-IV as the basis of practice and many organizations have not updated their internal documentation or electronic records. The main difference between the two is the multi-axial diagnosis system which was discontinued in the DSM-5.

The multiaxial diagnosis is a framework on five different axis, or perspectives, which provided nomenclature to a patient's unique presentation. Axis I and II describe mental health conditions; Axis III describe medical conditions that impacted the patient's plan of care; Axis IV describe psychosocial conditions; and Axis V provided a numerical scale, the Global Assessment of Functioning (GAF), which would be a barometer of mental health and could be used to objectively evaluate a patient's progress or regression in between evaluations.

The Axis I diagnosis are labeled Clinical Disorders, these are the kinds of disorders that one usually thinks about when considering mental health issues. Psychotic disorders (breaks from reality), such as Schizophrenia and mood disorders such as Major Depressive Disorder (MDD), Bipolar Disorder, and Generalized Anxiety Disorder (GAD) appear on the Axis I and we will discuss each of these individually as they compromise a very large percentage of the patients we see.

The Axis II diagnosis are reserved for Personality Disorders (PDs) and the Mental Retardation (MR) and Developmental Disability (DD) spectrum. PDs are maladaptive patterns of behavior and cognition which deviate markedly from those accepted by the patient's individual culture. It is often described as a patient's character, it is the way they think about themselves and others along with the way they act. It is believed that a person's personality is not fixed until adulthood so PDs may only be diagnosed after the age of 18. PDs in patient's under 18 are diagnosed separately and are placed on the Axis I; PDs will be addressed later in the primer. MR and DD are a group of diverse, chronic conditions that are due to mental or physical impairments. These are generally easy to diagnose early in a patient's lifespan and many require a diagnosis prior to age of 18. These include Down Syndrome, Fetal Alcohol Syndrome, as well as intellectual disabilities which is defined as anyone with an intelligence quotient (IQ) lower than 70.

Providers of mental health care vary in both their scope and practice. We will examine those who practice with a biomedical model, such as psychiatrists and psychiatric nurse practitioners, and those with a theoretical model such as psychologists and Licensed Clinical Social Workers (LCSW). We will discuss medication therapies along with the conditions they are generally used for and some of the treatment modalities that the theoretical model provider's concentrate on.

An increasingly alarming concern throughout healthcare and society at large is substance abuse. Mental Health issues and substance abuse often go hand-in-hand, frequently they are treated together. We will go through a brief overview of substance abuse later on.

The Psychiatric Consultation

The psychiatric consultation begins with the multiaxial diagnosis. The most frequently asked question is the difference between an Axis I and Axis II diagnosis. Axis I diagnosis tend to be episodic and treatable by psychiatric care, especially medication, while Axis II diagnosis are chronic conditions that tend to have no psychiatric care available (medications). While rarely mentioned in professional literature, the concept is well understood by medical professionals and the medical insurance industry – which will not pay for the inpatient treatment of a primary Axis II disorder. There is neither medication available to make an antisocial personality disorder a lawful member of society nor a medication which will grant IQ points to someone with an intellectual disorder. While there is a theoretical basis for a change in personality, it takes a concentrated effort on the part of the patient and much introspection – usually with the assistance of a psychologist or LCSW, generally on an outpatient basis.

The Axis III disorders are medical in nature and affect the plan of care for the patient. Medical conditions such as diabetes are of concern, especially in patients receiving medications which can promote weight gain. It is important for mental health providers to be aware of conditions that the patient may be taking medications for. Many psych meds have severe drug-drug interactions such as the antidepressant class of monoamine oxidase inhibitors (MAOIs) which are incompatible with virtually all other medications. Physical and mental limitations of conditions also impact the planning of our case and requires addressing. Additionally, some medical disorders masquerade as psychiatric disorders and when they are diagnosed or listed as a "rule-out" condition by the psychiatrist they should be added to the Axis III.

It's worth noting that there are many different physical conditions that either mimic or can be confused with mental illnesses. An unusual case was reported of a man who a head injury during a war and required surgery, including the addition of a metal plate in his head. One of his symptoms afterwards was a musical, auditory hallucination which waxed and waned in intensity. He was never troubled by it and he didn't report it until he travel to visit a son and suddenly started experiencing human voices instead of the musical hallucinations. Further review of his strange symptoms revealed that the metal plate was picking up radio waves and the man was "hearing" a frequency that played music in his home town but was talk radio in his son's town.

Ruling out medical conditions before diagnosing psychiatric conditions is paramount to the mental health clinician. Conditions such as delirium (rapid onset and usually reversible) can be confused with dementia (slow onset and irreversible, though progress may be slowed). Thyroid disorders frequently cause mood disturbances and anxiety. Anxiety is also a symptom of heart disease, diabetes, and multiple respiratory disorders.

The MSE

The heart of the psychiatric documentation is the MSE. It is the structured way we document a patient's current condition. The process is often referred to as the psychiatric interview. Even before we speak with the patient we assess their appearance and their movement, if possible. What kind of clothing are they wearing? Colorful or bizarre clothing may indicate a manic/hypomanic episode. Are they disheveled? Lack of self-care may indicate a depression or a negative symptom of schizophrenia. We look for signs and symptoms of ETOH or other substance abuse: is there track marks visible (from injectable drug use), malnutrition apparent, facial skin scabs, etc. The patient's attitude (cooperative, guarded, etc.) is noted as well as their behavior. Do they make eye contact? How was their gait? We describe any psychomotor agitation or retardation apparent. Agitation may be a sign of bipolar or a side-effect to a neuroleptic medication, which is serious and will be discussed in the section regarding antipsychotic medications.

A MSE includes documentation of a patient's **mood** and **affect**. Simply, mood is what a patient is feeling and affect is what a patient shows. The only way to know a patient's mood is to ask and we describe it in their terms. Their affect is what we observe, we label is according to how well it "agrees" with their mood and how expressive it is. A patient may tell you he is happy but his face looks flat or even depressed. We would document that affect, "…was incongruous with mood." The range of expression is noted, usually in terms of increasing range: flat, blunted, restricted, normal, and wide.

Evaluation of the patient's speech can provide us with insight into their condition. We note the rate (speed) and tone (both quality and strength) of the patient's speech, speech that is either retarded or agitated are diagnostically similar to their psychomotor counterparts. The content of their speech is assessed; constant repetition of the interviewer's speech (echolalia) and the creation of "new" words (neologisms) are indicative of altered thought content. Problems with speech, such as expressive as receptive aphasias, can point to a medical condition (cranial neoplasms or other neurological disorders) rather than a psychiatric one.

As the interview continues, the clinician evaluates the thought process of the patient in terms of its quantity, tempo, and coherence. Often a patient appears to be stumbling in their speech, trying to get all their thoughts out but unable to keep up. This racing speech is a strong symptom of bipolar. Other times patients can be difficult to interview, their thoughts go from subject to subject before returning to the original subject (**circumstantial**) or they continue to other subjects, unable to return to the original one (**tangential**). Sometimes the subject changes are quick and have no common thread, they are only linked to each other. These flights of ideas are indicative of the disorganized schizophrenic. The disorganization can become even more severe where sentence structure breaks down and it appears only near-random words are spoken, the word salad.

After the evaluation of the patient's speech and process, we examine the patient's thought content. Any perceptions of an altered reality are noted as a psychosis. These are mainly divided into false beliefs and hallucinations. False beliefs and other delusions are further categorized such as paranoid, grandiose, **erotomanic**, etc. It is important to understand the patient's cultural and socioeconomic background for reference as they may differ from the interviewer's and if culturally acceptable in the patient's realm it would not be considered a psychosis. Ruminations, thoughts which reoccur frequently and are troublesome to the patient, are noted, these are symptomatic of an obsessive or compulsive disorder.

Suicidal and homicidal thoughts or ideations are assessed. While often stated, it bears repeating that asking a patient if they wish to kill themselves does not plant the idea in their head. The specific question must also be asked, interviewers are sometimes tempted to soften the question by asking if the patient has any ideas of hurting themselves. To a deeply depressed person who is considering killing themselves, the act of suicide may not be considered hurtful. Instead, it is a release of pain – described to me by a suicidal patient as a way to, "… make the hurt stop." When considering safety risks for a patient it's prudent to ask both the questions of self-harm and the presence of any suicidal ideation. If ideation exists, it is imperative that the intent and any plans are assessed along with the means of acting on the plans. Similarly with homicidal ideation the questions specifically should be asked if the patient has any ideations of killing someone; if present then additional queries must be made as per suicidal thoughts.

There are legal requirements for any mental health professionals that become aware of specific homicidal ideation. The landmark **Tarasoff** case in California held that mental health professionals have a duty to protect individuals who are being threatened with bodily harm by a patient. Often called a "duty to warn", any threat towards an individual necessitates informing law enforcement and/or warning the intended victim.

Alterations in perception can be in the form of hallucinations and illusions. Illusions are misperceptions of reality and are not necessarily a psychotic symptom. Most people have had the experience of leaving a jacket or other clothing on a chair near a bed and then waking up and perceiving the clothing as a person standing near their bed. The clothing is misperceived as a person. A hallucination has no basis in reality and is always a psychotic symptom. Hallucinations can come from any sensory source: auditory, visual, tactile, gustatory, or olfactory but in psychiatry our main concern is auditory hallucinations which are the cardinal symptom of schizophrenia. The other hallucinations are diagnostic in that they point towards non-psychiatric disorders – which we will cover later.

The assessment and documentation of cognition begins simply with the patient's alertness and orientation. Next patient's memory is briefly assessed, both short-term and long-term memory. Serial 7s are often used, instructing the patient, "If we start from 100 and subtract seven, we get 93. Could you please subtract seven again and keep repeating that until I tell you to stop?" If the patient is **innumeric** one could ask the patient to spell, "world," and then spell it backwards. Long-term memory is assessed by asking questions about current or remote events, traditionally the current and previous presidents. Other questions about current and remote events may also be asked to assess a patient's fund of knowledge which would indicate a certain level of engagement or education. It is also worth noting if a patient's current fund of knowledge is incongruent with their level of education. Language functions should be assessed and noted if English is not the patient's first or native language. Executive functions are an indication of how well the patient integrates their knowledge with problems. It is often assessed by asking the patient to explain a proverb that is not too commonly used. "Could you explain to me what, 'Even monkeys fall from trees,' means?" A lower-functioning cognition, described as **concrete**, would answer akin to, "Sometimes monkeys climb up trees and fall down." A higher-functioning cognition, described as **abstract**, would answer something like, "Even an expert can fail at a task sometimes." Someone with an impaired or fractured cognition would provide an answer that is incomprehensible or has nothing to do with the proverb.

Lastly we provide an overview of the patient's insight and judgement. Insight is the ability to know the circumstances which surround the patient while judgement is what the patient does with that information. Similarly to mood and affect, insight and judgment may be incongruent. "I know that space aliens have poisoned my food so I have to go to the 7/11 to buy snacks," is an example of poor insight but good judgement. "I have bipolar disorder and I freak out when I don't take my meds but I don't feel like taking them," is an example of good insight and poor judgement.

Schizophrenia

Schizophrenia is generally considered the most debilitating of the MH illnesses. Its etymology is from the Greek meaning, "fractured thought". It is breaks with reality not, as sometimes portrayed in media, multiple personalities. Schizophrenia affects about one percent of the population, cross-culturally. One out of every 100 Americans, Kenyans, Chinese, etc. have schizophrenia. Not all MH disorders are cross-cultural, in that some disorders are only present in certain populations or geographic areas. Cross-cultural psych will be discussed later.

The clinical prognosis of a schizophrenic patient can be grim. There is an axiom of the rule of thirds where, "A third get better, a third stay the same, and a third get worse." On first presentation, schizophrenics are often misdiagnosed (the third that get better) and are later shown to be suffering from a mood disorder such bipolar disorder or a major depression with psychotic features or under the influence of a substance. Of the remaining, about half are stable and have episodic inpatient admissions for exacerbations of their symptoms. The other half descend into a severe and chronic psychosis and have limited functioning outside an institution.

The symptoms of schizophrenia are divided into positive symptoms and negative symptoms. Positive symptoms are simply those symptoms that are present in patients with schizophrenia while negative symptoms are presentations and behaviors that are present in non-schizophrenic individuals but absent from patients with schizophrenia.

Positive symptoms of schizophrenia include the cardinal schizophrenia symptom of auditory hallucinations. Commonly called "voices", auditory hallucinations are not experienced by patients as voices inside their heads. The hallucinations appear to them as an external voice, often as loud and clear as anyone speaking next to them. While older patients with schizophrenia understand that when clinicians ask them about "voices" we mean auditory hallucinations, younger patients may not. Rather than ask patients if they are hearing voices, a better question would be, "Have you ever had the experience of hearing someone talking to you when you were alone?"

The voices experienced by schizophrenics are usually unpleasant and sometimes tortuous. Sometimes they contain command hallucinations, which tell them to do something. It is important to note any command hallucinations which tell the patient to hurt themselves or anyone else. The voices may be a chorus, an individual, or conversations that may or may not address the patient.

If one would imagine a first presentation of an auditory hallucination, one may understand the genesis of delusion thought which often follows. If you were to imagine hearing a voice in the morning when alone in your bedroom, you would instinctively start looking for the source. Unable to find a source, the subject generally starts down one of two paths: the source is a powerful organization with the means to "bug" their bedroom (a government agency, a large corporation, or secret society); or paranormal/spiritual (God, angels, etc.) When the subject thinks that they are being targeted by an organization, they generally start forming paranoid delusions (the organization is "out to get me") and delusions of grandiosity ("I must be important if the KGB is targeting me.") Similarly, the subject thinking the auditory hallucinations are divine or spiritual starts forming religious delusions ("God has spoken to me, he told me what he wants me to do) and grandiosity often follows as well.

Negative symptoms include reduced social interaction and avoidance of others. While this may be from the disease process, it is certainly compounded by interactions that the patient has with others who do not share their experiences. "God talks to me. Doesn't he talk to you? Can't you hear him too?" Other negative symptoms include reduced affect, older schizophrenics often have a completely blunted affect. Anhedonia, the lack of pleasure in activities one once found enjoyable, is another common negative symptom.

Hallucinations and Diagnosis

Hallucinations can be diagnostic by their type. Barring any medical conditions, auditory hallucinations are the cardinal symptom of Schizophrenia. It is worth noting that a large number of people experience hypnogogic hallucinations – hallucinations which happen around the period the subject is falling asleep. These are completely normal and dissipate on being roused, subjects troubled by these should be reassured that they are not "going crazy". It is simply an early onset of the dream state.

Visual, olfactory, and gustatory hallucinations are generally neurological in origin. Any of these should be fully investigated and cleared by a neurologist before a psychiatric condition is considered. These are generally the hallmark of brain neoplasms or other masses compressing nerves. Only a very small percentage of MH patients claim they experience visual hallucinations. One condition of note is the Lewy Body dementia where the subjects experience so-called Lilliputian hallucinations, named after the characters from the novel *Gulliver's Travels*. These visual hallucinations appear in the periphery of the visual field as small characters that appear to be uninterested or do not interact with the subject, often described as "elves" or "fairies".

Tactile hallucinations are a strong indication of substance abuse. Generally they are caused by stimulants in active use or depressants in withdrawal. Most health care professionals are experienced with the methamphetamine abuser complaining of bugs crawling under their skin.

These subjects often pick at their skin during these paresthesias and have scabs or infections, particularly around their face – the famous "meth face". Likewise, most health care professionals are aware of the paresthesias described by those withdrawing from ETOH or opioids, "I've got spiders crawling all over my skin."

Antipsychotic Medication

Management of schizophrenia and other Axis I psychotic disorders is primarily pharmaceutical. Antipsychotic medication is available in two broad categories, the typicals and the atypicals. Typical medication includes the original antipsychotics Haldol (haloperidol) and Thorazine (chlropromazine). Typical antipsychotics, while generally very effective for psychotic symptom management, have some unpleasant side effects including sedation. Since they act on the brain's mesolimbic pathway, they also affect movement. It is very important for clinicians to assess and document a patient's baseline movement in order to monitor for changes. Commonly, the Abnormal Involuntary Movement Scale (AIMS) is completed – it is a standardized scale measuring potential side effects attributed to neuroleptics. These

Extrapyramidal Side Effects (EPS) often take the form of involuntary twitching of the index finger and thumb ("pill-rolling"), a rigid and staggering gait (parkinsonism), **dystonias** such as torticollis (involuntary stretching of the neck forward), and abnormal lip smacking and other buccal movements. As a whole, it is often described as the "Thorazine shuffle", which was seen in patients who were long-term recipients of chlorpromazine treatment. Symptoms generally resolve on discontinuation or dose reduction of the typical antipsychotic or when an anticholinergic such as Cogentin (benztropine) is added. If untreated, EPS can become permanent, symptoms remain even with the discontinuation of the neuroleptic. This condition is known Tardive Dyskinesia (TD) and can be thought of as an **iatrogenically**-induced Parkinson's. Because of the potential severity of adding a chronic disorder to the burden of a patient being treated with antipsychotics, the importance of regular monitoring of patient movement cannot be stressed enough.

Atypical medications such as Zyprexa (olanzapine) and Abilify (aripiprazole) are often less sedating but have different side effect profile. Atypicals are noted to generally cause weight gain, especially olanzapine. Even with patient education on nutrition and exercise, weight gain is usually seen. Patients with such weight gain are exposed to obvious additional health risks, most notably diabetes. Increased weight and blood glucose has been identified as metabolic syndrome, which is similar to TD (in that untreated EPS leads to TD, in effect "giving" the patient Parkinson's) in that metabolic syndrome may lead to an iatrogenically-induced diabetes. Atypicals also have the potential (but much reduced) to cause EPS and should also be monitored regularly for movement disorders. The atypical Clozaril (clozapine) is a special case which require monitoring of WBC as neutropenias have been observed. These patients are generally entered on a registry and require regular review as a condition of treatment with clozapine.

Major Depressive Disorder

One of the most common Axis I disorder is Major Depressive Disorder (MDD) which affect about seven percent of adults in the US. The two major diagnostic criteria for MDD is a depressed mood (which lasts most of the day, every day, for at least two weeks) and anhedonia in a similar time frame. MDD patients always require a suicide assessment, with every clinical encounter. It bears repeating that asking questions about killing themselves does not "plant the thought" in the patient's mind. It not uncommon for MDD patients to have suicidal ideation without intent or plan but they should be referred for further assessment to a MH provider.

Antidepressants

One biomedical theory of the cause of MDD is a lack of a specific neurotransmitter in the brain Serotonin (5-hydroxytryptamine) is believed to regulate mood, appetite, sleep, memory and sexual desire and function. Some brain cells produce serotonin and others uptake it, the amount of free serotonin in the CNS can be thought of as a "happy bath" for the brain. Therefore, the pharmacological goal is to increase serotonin levels, primarily by preventing its reuptake. Paxil (paroxetine) and Pexeva (paroxetine mesylate) are examples of selective serotonin reuptake inhibitors (SSRIs) commonly prescribed as first line antidepressants. The most common side effect is gastric distress (serotonin is actually most prevalent in the human gut, 90% of our supply is in the intestinal tract) which generally disappears within one to two weeks. The most common reason SSRIs are stopped by patients are sexual problems such as decreased libido, anorgasmia (the inability to achieve orgasm despite stimulation), or erectile dysfunctions. Patients should be encouraged to talk to their prescriber of antidepressants about these issues as decreasing doses or switching to another medication is often effective but patients tend to be embarrassed or attribute these problems to their MDD and not think it important to bring up.

There are additional classes of antidepressants which target other neurotransmitters and hormones. The serotonin and norepinephrine reuptake inhibitors (SNRIs) include Cymbalta (duloxetine) which has a similar side effect profile to the SSRIs with the exception of a decrease in the reports of sexual problems. The norepinephrine and dopamine reuptake inhibitors (NDRIs) include Wellbutrin/Zyban (bupropion hydrochloride). Both the SNRIs and NDRIs have a similar side effect profile to the SSRIs with the exception of an increase in the reports of anxiety and a decrease in the reports of sexual problems.

Atypical antidepressants have a nebulous method of action which is not well understood. Remeron (mirtazapine) and Desyrel (trazodone) are two examples. Remeron is noted for its ability to induce sleep and is generally prescribed for hs administration while trazodone is overwhelmingly sedating at therapeutic levels and generally only prescribed at lower doses as a hypnotic rather than as an antidepressant.

The tricyclic antidepressants, such as Tofranil (imipramine) and Pamelor (nortiptyline), are often the second-line prescribed therapeutic agents when one of the newer generation anti-depressants have failed the patient. Tricyclics are noted for their ability to assist with issues of chronic pain and are often prescribed by medical providers for that indication. Patients on tricyclics require especially close monitoring of suicidal ideation as the lethal overdose potential of these medications is quite high.

One of the oldest categories of antidepressants is the monoamine oxidase inhibitors (MAOIs) such as Nardil (phenelzine). It's also the only class with a non-oral means of administration available, Emsam (selegiline) is available as a transdermal patch. The MAOIs require the patient to adhere to a strict tyramine-free diet and thus require intensive education of foods that include tyramine including many cheeses, aged meat, tap or home-brewed beer, soy products, and many more. MAOIs are incompatible with virtually all medications, the last line of almost every voice over heard during a drug commercial on television is, "Do not take within two weeks of taking an MAOI." MAOIs are generally only prescribed as a last try after failure of all other drug classes and are contraindicated in most patients that have chronic medical conditions requiring pharmacological treatment.

Antidepressant discontinuation syndrome is a condition that may occur when antidepressants, particularly of the serotonin reuptake inhibitor classes (SSRIs and SNRIs), are abruptly discontinued or have large decreases in dose. Symptoms include flu-like symptoms and disturbances in the patient's sleep, movement, mood, and cognition. Some patient's complain of feeling electric-shocks in the brain, frequently described as, "brain zaps". While these symptoms are transient and generally dissipate within a month, they can be alleviated by reintroduction of the antidepressant or titrating more slowly the dose reduction. Reintroduction of the antidepressant generally removes all symptoms within one day.

It is important to educate patients about the timeframes for antidepressant effects. Beyond the placebo effect of beginning an antidepressant, the first effects of treatment are generally not noticed for one to two weeks and full effects not until four to six weeks. Generally, antidepressants are started on the lowest dose possible and titrated week by week (to monitor for side effects) until the usual dose is achieved. Then, usually after a month to six weeks, the dose may be titrated further to achieve the maximum therapeutic benefit.

Bipolar Disorder

Bipolar disorder, formerly Manic Depression, is episodic periods of mania and depression. Mania can be manifested by inflated self-esteem or grandiosity, often to a delusional point, "I am in talks with a major motion picture studio to make a movie about my life." A marked decrease in the need for sleep is usually apparent along with increased psychomotor agitation. Additionally, there is greatly increased goal-oriented activity, often to the point of absurdity such as going to a car dealership and attempting to buy, "…every car on the lot. I want them all." During manic episodes, patients often are hyper verbal or display pressured speech. These patients often have unique and colorful attire, sometimes quite bizarre. It is not unusual for women to use brightly colored lipstick, extending a centimeter or more beyond their lips, and use the same lipstick to mark other areas of their face with designs or symbols. Mania also often drives patients to engage in high-risk activities such as massive and unnecessary spending sprees and sexual promiscuity. Large amounts of debt and a history of multiple sexually transmitted diseases can be indicative of previous manic episodes. It is important to note any substance abuse history prior to considering a diagnosis of bipolar disorder as many of these, especially stimulant, can mimic the effects of mania.

In describing the bipolar disorder cycles, diagrams of sine waves are often shown. This is misleading as the symptom pattern of patients rarely follow regular patterns. There can be successive periods of mania with differing intervals before a depressive period. The cycles are also weeks in duration, not days or hours. A patient who says they feel depressed in the morning but manic in the evening would indicate more a problem on the Axis II than in the realm of a mood disorder like bipolar.

When the patient is departing from **euthymia** and begins to climb the cycle towards mania, they enter a condition known as hypomania. **Hypomania**, similar to mania but on a much reduced scale, can be a period of greater productivity and creativity for patients. Many highly successful artists, inventors, businessmen, etc. are able to live as hypomanics.

Pharmacological Treatment for Bipolar Disorder

Pharmacological treatment of bipolar medication is usually one of the mood stabilizers. Lithium has a long history of treating bipolar disorder. It requires frequent blood draws for level titration until it is within the therapeutic range. The range is quite narrow and it can be a challenge for patients to remain within the target range. In warmer climates, dehydration can push the lithium patient into lithium toxicity, causing nausea, vomiting, diarrhea, muscle weakness, tremor, blurred vision, and tinnitus.

Valproic acid and its derivatives (Depakote and Depakene) are a more recent addition to the historical treatment of bipolar. This have a much wider therapeutic range and require less blood monitoring. They are also safer in overdoses than Lithium.

In the manic phase, patients are often prescribed antipsychotics to assist with behavioral control and reduction in delusional though. The sedating properties of the typical antipsychotics are often considered beneficial to manic patients during their episodes of mania. Many atypical antipsychotic drug manufacturers market their products as adjunctive treatments (for use every day, not just during manic phases) for bipolar disorder and other mood disorders but many clinicians have raised concerns over polypharmacy within psychiatry and will not prescribe adjunctive antipsychotics. The Joint Commission also monitors psychiatric polypharmacy, especially more than one **neuroleptic**.

During depressive phases, many clinicians provide antidepressant therapy. Antidepressant use in diagnosed bipolar patients need to be carefully monitored as there is the possibility that prolonged use may push the patient into a manic episode. This risk of potential **activation** can be reduced by titrating and then discontinuing the antidepressant when euthymia is achieved.

Benzodiazepines

Drug	Dose Equivalents (mg)	Half Life (hrs)	Usual Adult Daily Dosage (mg/day)
Chlordiazepoxide (Librium)	10	100	15-100
Diazepam (Valium)	5	100	2-60
Flurazepam (Dalmane)	5	100	15-30
Clonazepam (Clonopin)	0.5	100	.5-10
Lorazepam (Ativan)	1	15	2-6
Temazepam (Resoril)	5	11	16-30
Oxazepam (Serax)	15	8	30-120
Alprazolam (Xanax)	0.25	12	.5-6

Triazolam (Halcion)	0.1	2	.125-.25
Estazolam (ProSom)	0.33	17	1-2

Benzodiazepines, often shortened to simply benzos, are often referred to as the "Pams" for their drug name suffix such as diazepam, lorazepam, and clonazepam. These medications have a very strong **anxiolytic** and sedative effect. They are commonly used for anxiety disorders and the sedation of agitated patients, hence they are often prescribed, for short-term usage, for those in a current manic cycle for symptomatic management. Benzodiazepines have a very strong potential for addiction and abuse. For any patient, regular usage should be for periods of less than two weeks. Usage in chronic conditions like anxiety should only be on a PRN basis; any consistent usage for two weeks or more should be tapered off to avoid the withdrawal effects of abrupt discontinuation. The addiction potential increases inversely with the medication's half-life. Valium (diazepam) and Librium (diazepam) have very long half-lives (about 100 hours) and are actually used to prevent withdrawal symptoms in the detoxification of patients addicted to depressants like ETOH. Xanax (alprazolam) and Ativan (lorazepam) have very short half-lives (12 and 15 hours respectively) and are notoriously difficult medications to withdraw from.

Generalized Anxiety Disorder

Generalized anxiety disorder (GAD) is the most frequent diagnosis on the anxiety spectrum. Primarily manifested as excessive anxiety and/or worry that is difficult for the patient to control, it also has a somatic component of any combination of the following: restlessness, feeling keyed up or on edge; easily fatigued; difficulty concentrating or mind going blank; irritability, muscle tension; and sleep disturbance.

Pharmacological treatment for GAD is often achieved with the short-term usage of benzodiazepines; non-benzo anxiolytics such as BuSpar (buspirone); antidepressants (particularly the SSRI class); antihistamines such as Vistaril (hydroxyzine); and beta blockers such as propranolol. It is interesting to note that patients who are naïve to benzos have a much greater response to non-benzo anxiolytics. Additionally, the beta blockers are particularly effective to assist with the GAD's complaint of "feelings of impending doom" and for those who suffer from performance anxiety.

Personality Disorders

The Axis II disorders are compromised of the mental retardation / developmental disability spectrum and the personality disorders. The MR/DD disorders are beyond the scope of this primer; we will concentrate on the different disorders of personality. Little discussion of treatment options will be offered; pharmaceutical management may occur for symptomatic relief but is often ineffective. Personality disorders cannot be "cured" by psychiatric care, this requires both a desire on the patient's part to modify their personality or character and the tools to do so. Different therapeutic treatment modalities are available from psychologists, clinical social workers, and other counselors – we will discuss them later.

Personality disorders (PDs) are categorized into three different clusters: cluster A (the "mad", in the sense they appear psychotic), cluster B (the "bad", in the difficulties their actions cause), and cluster C (the "sad", personalities that appear as mood disorders). Specifically cluster B disorders can cause significant tribulations in clinical interactions, mental health professionals often use the term in referencing patients to indicate less a diagnosis but more that the patient is difficult to work with or causes problems, "Mr. Jones, a real cluster B, has been admitted today."

Cluster A Personality Disorders "The Mad"

Cluster A disorders are composed of the paranoid personality disorder, the schizoid personality disorder, and the schizotypal personality disorder. Each of these disorders contain signs and symptoms that appear, or are, psychotic but the genesis of these psychosis is in their character, not a disease process like schizophrenia. For their similarity to patients with psychotic axis I disorders, this cluster is referred to as the "mad". It is worth noting that these psychotic symptoms are rarely alleviated with the introduction of antipsychotic medications.

The Paranoid PD is a pattern of distrust and suspiciousness such that others' motives are interpreted as malevolent. It begins by early childhood, is present in a variety of contexts, and does not occur during the course of schizophrenia, or other Axis I disorders and medical conditions (including substance abuse) have been ruled out. These patients are difficult to interview, believing their experiences are, "…not anybody's business." They are often jealous of their partner's fidelity, without any basis, and any injuries or slights, no matter how minor, will often provoke major feelings of hostility which will persist for a very long time. Offers of assistance or help will often be viewed as an attack, "You don't think I can do this myself?"

The Schizoid PD is a pervasive pattern of detachment from social relationships and a restricted range of expression in a variety of contexts. The signs and symptoms appear very much like the negative symptoms of schizophrenia but lack any positive ones. It begins by early childhood and does not occur during the course of schizophrenia, autism, or other Axis I disorders and medical conditions (including substance abuse) have been ruled out. These patients appear to lack a desire for intimacy, seem indifferent to any opportunity to develop close relationships, and usually do not derive any positive feelings from being part of a social group or family. Frequently they are described as "loners" by themselves and others.

The Schizotypal PD is a pervasive pattern of social and interpersonal deficits marked by acute discomfort with, and diminished capacity for, close relationships and cognitive or perceptual distortions along with eccentricities in behavior. Their odd beliefs (usually supernatural or extraterrestrial) and strange behavior (the traditional tin foil hat, "…to block out the signals the aliens are sending me) make meaningful relationships difficult and they often have few friends and little contact with family other than first-degree relations. Obviously a clinician needs to rule out schizophrenia and other Axis I disorder before a schizotypal PD can be identified. A belief that an alien entity can send a signal to their brain is very different from hearing alien voices and trying to overcome that with a hat lined with tinfoil.

Cluster B Personality Disorders "The Bad"

The Cluster B personality disorders are characterized by intense difficulties in understanding or conforming to the norms of interpersonal interaction. They include the antisocial PD, the borderline PD, the histrionic PD, and the narcissistic PD. This cluster causes the most disruption to the clinic or therapeutic milieu and they are often referred to as the, "bad".

The Antisocial PD is a pervasive pattern of disregard for, and violation of, the rights of others that begins during childhood or early adolescence and continues on into childhood. Sometimes antisocial PD is described as psychopathy or sociopathy. The central features of this PD is deceit and manipulation, thus these patients are poor historians and will require collateral information from other sources to paint a good clinical photo. Usually these patients have little to no empathy for others and see other people merely as a vehicle to supply their needs and wants. They draw from their own experience in manipulating others in encounters. A common scene in an inpatient setting is as follows:

"Wow, nurse. You sure are pretty today. Love those scrubs. Can I have a cigarette?"

If the request is refused, "Sorry, but it's not time yet," the antisocial PD switches to another tactic.

"Oh. Well. I saw you drive in today. You're driving a green Honda Civic, right? Would be a shame if something happened to it. Or you. Can I have a cigarette?"

The patient is using a **veiled threat** to attempt to get what they want. It is important to address this, bearing in mind immediate staff safety. Threats of any kind, even couched, should be assessed and explained to the patient as unacceptable, preferably with multiple staff members in attendance, and then brought up during the **interdisciplinary treatment team** (IDTT). In this scenario the nurse again denies the request.

"Yeah, well f___ you. I'm gonna kill you." Patients with antisocial PD rarely have impulse control and will often quickly resort to violent threats (raising fists, etc.) or actual violence with little warning.

The Borderline PD is essentially a pervasive pattern of instability of interpersonal relationships, self-image, and affects couples with marked impulsivity that begins by early adulthood. The etymology for the term borderline comes from early versions of categorizing mental health disorders (DSM II), prior to the multiaxial system. Disorders were put into two categories, the psychotics (those patients who break from reality such as schizophrenia) and the neurotics (those with chronic distress such as depression). Clinicians noted that there was a class of neurotics who, when in crisis, appeared to straddle or cross over into psychosis. They were said to have been on the "borderline" of neurosis and psychosis and the clinical term stuck. Patients with borderline PD make frantic efforts to avoid real or imagined abandonment. They frequently demonstrate "help-seeking, help-rejecting" behaviors wherein they seek out treatment or help with the immense void they feel within themselves but then quickly leave treatment before they get "dropped". These patients also over-inflate the importance of some of their relationships, believing that superficial relations with others are actually much deeper than they actually are. In crisis, typically when the patient feels abandoned such as the end of a relationship, they may experience some paranoid delusions or **disassociative** symptoms such as **depersonalization**. Disassociative symptoms are disorders that involve a disconnection between cognition, memories, actions, and identity. Some may complain of amnesia, often they claim **fugue**-like states where they walk around in a "fog" or "on autopilot" and then resume normal activities and are unaware of what they did during the fugue.

Even without any psychological treatment, patients with borderline PD tend to have greater vocational and relational stability over time beginning in their late 30s to early 40s. Over half of all diagnosed borderline PDs no longer meet diagnostic criteria for the disorder after 10 years.

The Histrionic PD is marked by a pattern of pervasive and excessive emotionality and attention-seeking behavior. Unhappy if they are not the center of attention, these patients generally try to get positive attention from those around them but will seek out negative attention in addition to or to supplement missing positive attention. Often inappropriately seductive or sexually provocative, they spend an inordinate amount of time, energy, and money on clothing and grooming. They are especially noted for considering casual acquaintances or health providers as close friends even after just a first or second meeting, they will frequently want to be on first name basis with treating physicians and providers.

The Narcissistic PD is similar to the histrionic but only positive attention is sought. These patients demonstrate a pervasive pattern of grandiosity, need for admiration, and lack of empathy for others. By over-estimating their abilities and inflating their accomplishments, they expect admiration and praise from others and may be perplexed or even angry why it is not forthcoming. They may seek out special privileges or extra resources they believe they are entitled to because they are so special and then become angry when denied.

Narcissistic PD is often associated with **anorexia nervosa** and other eating disorders and has a high correlation with substance abuse disorders, specifically cocaine. These patients also have special difficulties adjusting to the onset of physical and vocational limitations that are inherent in the aging process.

Cluster C Personality Disorders "The Sad"

The cluster C disorders appears superficially similar to mood disorders on the axis I except the genesis of their presentation is their personality disorder. This cluster is often referred to as the, "sad". Similarly to cluster A disorders, patients in the cluster C disorders do not typically respond to antidepressants, or they respond atypically such as therapeutic benefits seen immediately after taking, suggesting a placebo response. The cluster C patients include the avoidant PD, the dependent PD, the obsessive-compulsive PD, and the depressive PD.

The Avoidant PD is a pervasive pattern of social inhibition, feelings of inadequacy, and hypersensitivity to negative evaluation. These patients typically avoid work activities that that involve significant interpersonal contact because of fears of criticism and rejection. They also tend to avoid promotional opportunities because of the perceived fears of conflict. In terms of friends, these individuals tend to avoid making new friends unless they are complete certain they will be liked and accepted without criticism. They tend to be shy and reserved and display a very low threshold for detecting criticism and rejection. These patients often have a very restricted lifestyle, fearful of taking personal risks or engaging in new activities.

The Dependent PD is a pervasive and excessive pattern of needing to be taken care of. They display submissive and "clingy" behavior along with fears of separation. These patients have great difficulty making everyday decisions (what colour clothing to wear, what do to about lunch, etc.) unless they have direction and reassurance from others. They are extremely passive and seek out parental or spousal direction for all major decisions such as where to live and career choices. Individuals with dependent PD will be much stressed when they perceive they are alone, any loss of a caregiver or relationship will generally drive them to seek out a replacement quickly and indiscriminately.

The Obsessive-Compulsive PD (OCPD)

is a preoccupation with orderliness, perfectionism coupled with mental and interpersonal control. The expression, "It's my way or the highway," was likely coined by an OCPD. This contrasts with the obsessive compulsive disorder (OCD), which is an axis II disorder. OCD is marked by rituals such as performing repetitive tasks specific amounts of time (such as turning on and off a light switch) and **ruminations** that are unpleasant and intrusive, such as imagining the home stove is on and having to leave work to check – even though they haven't used the stove recently.

OCPD patients attempt to make a sense of control over excessive and painstaking attention to rules, lists, schedules, and trivial details. Often oblivious to the fact that this can annoy others for the delays and inconveniences, they often are unable to complete projects as they spend inordinate amounts of time ensuring that every detail is perfect. These patients often display excessive devotion to work and productivity to the point where they limit leisure time and friendships, even when there is no economic necessity to do so. These individuals tend to be excessively conscientious, scrupulous, and demonstrate inflexibility in matters of morality, ethics, and values and expect the same of others. OCPD patients tend to be unable to discard worn-out or worthless items, even when there is no sentimental value attached to the object; they will often admit to being "pack rats". These patients often have limited ability to delegate tasks to others, demonstrating extreme stubbornness and declaring, "Things have to be done my way," and display irritation and anger if alternative methods are proposed. Some individuals display miserly or stingy behaviours and live far below their means, often in anticipation of a major catastrophe.

The Depressive PD diagnosis has been added, moved, and removed frequently in different revisions of the DSM. Currently, in DSM 5, it is diagnosed as dysthymic disorder or other specified personality disorder. The depressive PD patient's mood is dominated by dejection, gloominess, cheerlessness, joylessness and unhappiness. Think of the Disney character Eeyore. These patients are self-critical, self-blaming, and often regards others similarly by being negative and judgmental towards them as well. They are very pessimistic and prone towards feeling guilty or remorseful.

Mental Health Providers

The mental health providers one frequently encounters are divided into two groups, those that are trained in the biomedical model and those that follow the theoretical model. Psychiatrists are licensed physicians (MD) who have completed an additional four or five year residency in psychiatry. Psychiatric and mental health nurse practitioners (NP) are at least graduate-level trained nurses whose program of study was a psychiatric and mental health NP program or has completed an additional program to enable national certification. These providers primarily focus on mental health diagnosis and the exclusion of medical causes along with the pharmacological management of mental health illnesses. While some of these providers have training and experience in traditional therapies ("Talk" therapy) it is increasingly rare.

Clinical psychologists have graduated from a doctoral program in psychology and have pursued additional clinical experience for licensing. These providers focus on psychological testing (which includes intelligence testing) and in individual and group therapies. In some states they can apply for prescriptive authority for psychiatric medication, generally under the supervision of a physician.

Treatment Modalities

There are many different types of therapeutic modalities which can be of benefit to the patient with a mental health issue. Counselling is a broad category of one-on-one therapy, generally it either targets symptoms experienced by the patient or increases their self-awareness and insight. Cognitive behavioural therapy (CBT) concentrates on developing coping strategies by having patients understand the relation between thoughts, feelings, and behaviours; by modifying their own thoughts they can then change the way they feel and act. Psychotherapy is a lengthy process where the therapist guides the patient in understanding subconscious reasons for their feelings and actions and then confronting them in order to change the way they feel and act. Group therapy has patients together and uses a combination of other therapeutic methods to let them all share the experience and is particularly useful for

psychoeducation. Interpersonal therapy focuses on resolving interpersonal problems and symptomatic recovery. Mindful-based therapy, originally developed as a relapse-prevention for depression, concentrates on minimizing reaction to negative stimuli, instead accepting and observing them without judgement.

Substance abuse treatment is generally composed of three phases. The detoxification (detox) period is generally one to weeks of the medical management of withdrawal signs and symptoms. The rehabilitation phase is generally one to three months of inpatient or outpatient therapy where the patient is given coping mechanisms for achieving a substance-free lifestyle. In sobriety maintenance, which is ongoing and may continue with the patient their whole life, the patient uses individual and/or group therapies to continue to develop coping strategies for substance abstinence and support for their sobriety. Alcoholics Anonymous and Narcotics Anonymous are some traditional sobriety maintenance programs that are faith-based. Increasingly, non-faith-based programs such as SMART recovery, are being offered.

Cross Cultural Psychiatry

Vital to the diagnostic and treatment phases for all mental health patients is the provider's ability to be culturally competent. Symptoms which may be indicative of psychosis in one individual would not be in another whose culture where the symptom is considered normal or even expected. The provider must consider the patient's ethnic background, country of origin, religion, etc. in order to provide a diagnostic formulation. Interviews with friends and family, as corroborative information, is especially useful.

Consider a religious group such as the Pentacostalists who practice glossolalia (speaking in tongues) and demonstrate pseudo seizures during their services. Members are expected and encouraged to demonstrate these behaviors, these should not be considered psychiatric symptoms.

Some mental disorders are trans-cultural, in that they are observed in every geographic area – such, as we have seen, in schizophrenia. There are also some disorders that are unique to certain regions or cultural populations, these disorders may fit somewhat into the DSM diagnostic spectrum but one should be aware of other mental health diagnostic systems that exist. An example is the Chinese Classification of Mental Disorders (CCMD). An example of a CCMD diagnosis is *Qigong Deviation* (Psychosis) where a patient becomes psychotic after or during practice of *qigong* – a system of meditation and movement. I once met, in an American emergency room, a patient who appeared to be the textbook definition of Qigong Psychosis. While we labeled him a schizophrenic, we noted in our consultation that the treatment team should consider the cultural impacts towards this patient while formulating their care.

Running amok is a syndrome originating in Malaysia/Indonesia where an individual would suddenly attack people and/or objects, often after a period of brooding or isolation. The cultural belief is that the person is possessed by a malevolent spirit and that the individual, who often recounts they have no memory of the event. A DSM diagnosis would probably be either on the bipolar spectrum or cluster C PD – most probably antisocial PD.

Koro, a syndrome specific to the Pacific Rim but appearing now in Africa and Europe is the fixed delusion that one's genitalia or breasts are shrinking, often also including the belief that the sufferer will die when their genitals have disappeared. This causes enormous distress and sufferers will often go to extreme lengths to prevent further shrinkage (despite a lack of any objective changes) such as inserting metal pins or attaching strings to anchor themselves.

Resources

1-800-273-8255

National Suicide Prevention Lifeline

www.psychiatry.org/psychiatrists/practice/dsm

The American Psychiatric Association's website for the DSM

www.smartrecovery.org

A non-faith-based substance abuse recovery program

www.youtube.com/watch?v=0vvU-Ajwbok

An excellent simulation of auditory hallucinations

Mental Health Terms

Ψ The Greek letter Psi. Common shorthand for "psych". Seen in charting as "Ψ pt" or "r/o Ψ" to refer a psychiatric patient or a patient where a psychiatric disorder is suspected. Also ΨMD or ΨRN to refer to a psychiatrist or psychiatric nurse.

Abstract thinking The ability to think about objects, principles, and ideas that are not physically present. It is related to symbolic thinking, which uses the substitution of a symbol for an object or idea. Examples include: using metaphors and analogies; understanding relationships between verbal and non-verbal ideas; and reasoning, such as using critical thinking, the scientific method, and other approaches to reasoning through problems.

Activation A cluster of symptoms of excessive emotional arousal, sometimes progressing to mania, caused by antidepressant use, especially in the SSRI class.

Affect The experience of feeling or emotion. In mental health, it refers to affect display, which is facial, vocal, and gestural behavior that serves as an indicator of mood. In other words, mood is how the subjects feels while affect is what they show.

Anorexia nervosa Often referred to simply as anorexia, it is an eating and mental health disorder characterized by low weight, fear of gaining weight, and a strong desire to be thin, resulting in food restriction. Many people with anorexia see themselves as overweight even though they are in fact underweight. If asked they usually deny they have a problem with low weight. Often they weigh themselves frequently, eat only small amounts, and only eat certain foods. Some will exercise excessively, force themselves to vomit, or use laxatives to produce weight loss. Complications may include osteoporosis, infertility and heart damage, among others. Women will often stop having menstrual periods.

Antidepressant discontinuation syndrome A condition that can occur following the interruption, dose reduction, or discontinuation of antidepressant drugs, including selective serotonin re-uptake inhibitors (SSRIs) or serotonin–norepinephrine reuptake inhibitors (SNRIs). The symptoms can include flu-like symptoms and disturbances in sleep, senses, movement, mood, and thinking. In some cases, symptoms may be mild, short-lived, and resolve without treatment. More severe cases may only be successfully treated by reintroduction of the drug, provided reintroduction is done in a timely fashion. Symptoms, including tardive akathisia, and Post SSRI Sexual Dysfunction (PSSD) may persist for months to years.

Anxiolytic (also antipanic or antianxiety agent) A medication or other intervention that inhibits anxiety. This effect is in contrast to anxiogenic agents, which increase anxiety. Together these categories of psychoactive compounds or interventions may be referred to as anxiotropic compounds or agents. Some recreational drugs such as alcohol (also known formally as ethanol) induce anxiolysis initially; however, studies show that many of these drugs are anxiogenic. Anxiolytic medications have been used for the treatment of anxiety disorder and its related psychological and physical symptoms.

Circumstantial speech The result of a non-linear thought pattern. It occurs when the focus of a conversation drifts, but often comes back to the point. In circumstantiality, apparently unnecessary details and seemingly irrelevant remarks cause a delay in getting to the point.

Concrete thinking Literal thinking that is focused on the physical world. It is the opposite of abstract thinking. People engaged in concrete thinking are focused on facts in the here and now, physical objects, and literal definitions. The term "concrete thinking" is, ironically, a metaphor (and a metaphor is a type of abstract thinking); concrete is a hard, physical substance and concrete thinking is focused on literal–and often physical–facts. A person who thinks only in concrete terms might think that the term "concrete thinking" means thinking literally about concrete.

Diagnostic and Statistical Manual (DSM) Published by the American Psychiatric Association (APA), it offers a common language and standard criteria for the classification of mental disorders. It is used, or relied upon, by clinicians, researchers, psychiatric drug regulation agencies, health insurance companies, pharmaceutical companies, the legal system, and policy makers together with alternatives such as the ICD-10 Classification of Mental and Behavioural Disorders, produced by the WHO. The DSM is now in its fifth edition, the

DSM-5, published on May 18, 2013. The DSM evolved from systems for collecting census and psychiatric hospital statistics, and from a United States Army manual. Revisions since its first publication in 1952 have incrementally added to the total number of mental disorders, although also removing those no longer considered to be mental disorders.

Dissociation A wide array of experiences from mild detachment from immediate surroundings to more severe detachment from physical and emotional experiences. The major characteristic of all dissociative phenomena involves a detachment from reality, rather than a loss of reality as in psychosis. Dissociation is commonly displayed on a continuum. In mild cases, dissociation can be regarded as a coping mechanism or defense mechanisms in seeking to master, minimize or tolerate stress – including boredom or conflict. At the nonpathological end of the continuum, dissociation describes common events such as daydreaming. Further along the continuum are more pathological dissociations: a sense that self or the world is unreal (depersonalization and derealization); a loss of memory (amnesia); forgetting identity or assuming a new self (fugue);

and fragmentation of identity or self into separate streams of consciousness (dissociative identity disorder, formerly termed multiple personality disorder.

Dystonia A neurological movement disorder syndrome in which sustained or repetitive muscle contractions result in twisting and repetitive movements or abnormal fixed postures. The movements may resemble a tremor. Dystonia is often intensified or exacerbated by physical activity, and symptoms may progress into adjacent muscles.

Euthymia A normal, tranquil mental state or mood. It is often used to describe a stable mental state or mood in those affected with bipolar disorder that is neither manic nor depressive, yet is distinguishable from healthy controls. Euthymia is also used to describe the "baseline" of other cyclic mood disorders like major depressive disorder (MDD) and narcissistic personality disorder (NPD). This state is the goal of psychiatric and psychological interventions.

Erotomania A type of delusional disorder where the affected person believes that another person is in love with him or her. This belief is usually applied to someone with higher status or a famous person, but can also be applied to a complete stranger. Erotomanic delusions often occur in patients with schizophrenia and other psychotic disorders, but can also occur during a manic episode in the context of bipolar I disorder. During an erotomanic delusion, the patient believes that a secret admirer is declaring his or her affection for the patient, often by special glances, signals, telepathy, or messages through the media. Usually the patient then returns the perceived affection by means of letters, phone calls, gifts, and visits to the unwitting recipient. Even though these advances are unexpected and often unwanted, any denial of affection by the object of this delusional love is dismissed by the patient as a ploy to conceal the forbidden love from the rest of the world.

Extrapyramidal Side Effects Side effects from antipsychotic medications including acute dyskinesias and dystonic reactions, tardive dyskinesia, Parkinsonism, akinesia, akathisia, and neuroleptic malignant syndrome. Extrapyramidal symptoms are caused by dopamine blockade or depletion in the basal ganglia.

Fugue or dissociative fugue A dissociative disorder and a rare psychiatric disorder characterized by reversible amnesia for personal identity, including the memories, personality, and other identifying characteristics of individuality. The state can last days, months or longer. Dissociative fugue usually involves unplanned travel or wandering, and is sometimes accompanied by the establishment of a new identity. It is a facet of dissociative amnesia, according to the DSM 5. After recovery from a fugue state previous memories usually return intact, and further treatment is unnecessary. Additionally, an episode of fugue is not characterized as attributable to a psychiatric disorder if it can be related to the ingestion of psychotropic substances, to physical trauma, to a general medical condition, or to dissociative identity disorder,[clarification needed] delirium, or dementia. Fugues are precipitated by a series of long-term traumatic episodes. It is most commonly associated with childhood victims of sexual abuse who learn over time to dissociate memory of the abuse (dissociative amnesia).

Hypomania (literally "under mania" or "less than mania") A mood state characterized by persistent disinhibition and elevation (euphoria). It may involve irritation, but less severely than full mania. According to DSM 5 criteria, hypomania is distinct from mania in that there is no significant functional impairment; mania, by DSM 5 definition, does include significant functional impairment and may have psychotic features. Characteristic behaviors of persons experiencing hypomania are a notable decrease in the need for sleep, an overall increase in energy, unusual behaviors and actions, and a markedly distinctive increase in talkativeness and confidence, commonly exhibited with a flight of creative ideas. Other symptoms related to this may include feelings of grandiosity, distractibility, and hypersexuality. While hypomanic behavior often generates productivity and excitement, it can become troublesome if the subject engages in risky or otherwise inadvisable behaviors, and/or the symptoms manifest themselves in trouble with everyday life events. When manic episodes are separated into stages of a progression according to symptomatic severity and associated features, hypomania constitutes the first stage of the syndrome, wherein the cardinal features (euphoria or heightened irritability, pressure of speech and activity, increased energy, decreased need for sleep, and flight of ideas) are most plainly evident.

Iatrogenesis (from the Greek for "brought forth by the healer") Any effect on a person, resulting from any activity of one or more persons acting as healthcare professionals or promoting products or services as beneficial to health, that does not support a goal of the person affected. Some iatrogenic effects are clearly defined and easily recognized, such as a complication following a surgical procedure (e.g., lymphedema as a result of breast cancer surgery). Less obvious ones, such as complex drug interactions, may require significant investigation to identify. Consensus limits use of "iatrogenesis" to adverse effects, possibly including, broadly, all adverse unforeseen outcomes resulting from medication or other medical treatment or intervention.

Innumeracy The inability to reason and to apply simple numerical concepts. Basic numeracy skills consist of comprehending fundamental arithmetic concepts like addition, subtraction, multiplication, and division. For example, if one can understand simple mathematical equations such as, $2 + 2 = 4$, then one would be considered possessing at least basic numeric knowledge.

Interdisciplinary Treatment Team (IDTT) A patient-focused treatment team usually comprised of a treating mental health provider, a social worker, and nurse who meet regularly to monitor a patient's progress and evaluate changes needed to the plan of care.

Mental Status Exam The clinical assessment process in psychiatric practice. It is a structured way of observing and describing a patient's psychological functioning at a given point in time, under the domains of appearance, attitude, behavior, mood, and affect, speech, thought process, thought content, perception, cognition, insight, and judgment. The purpose of the MSE is to obtain a comprehensive cross-sectional description of the patient's mental state, which, when combined with the biographical and historical information of the psychiatric history, allows the clinician to make an accurate diagnosis and formulation, which are required for coherent treatment planning. The MSE is not to be confused with the Mini–Mental State Examination (MMSE), which is a brief neuro-psychological screening test for dementia.

Mood An emotional state. In contrast to emotions, feelings, or affects, moods are less specific, less intense and less likely to be provoked or instantiated by a particular stimulus or event. Moods are typically described as having either a positive or negative valence. In other words, people usually talk about being in a good mood or a bad mood. Mood also differs from temperament or personality traits which are even longer-lasting. Nevertheless, personality traits such as optimism and neuroticism predispose certain types of moods. Long term disturbances of mood such as clinical depression and bipolar disorder are considered mood disorders. Mood is an internal, subjective state but it often can be inferred from posture and other behaviors.

Neuroleptic An antipsychotic medication. Formally called a major tranquilizer to distinguish from the minor tranquilizers (benzodiazepines).

Psychoeducation An evidence-based therapeutic intervention for patients and their loved ones that provides information and support to better understand and cope with illness.

Psychoeducation is most often associated with serious mental illness, including dementia, schizophrenia, clinical depression, anxiety disorders, psychotic illnesses, eating disorders, personality disorders and autism, although the term has also been used for programs that address physical illnesses, such as cancer. Psychoeducation offered to patients and family members teaches problem-solving and communication skills and provides education and resources in an empathetic and supportive environment.

Rumination Repetitive thinking about a thought or a problem without completion. The subject is generally aware that the thought pattern is abnormal and intrusive and finds it unwelcome.

Tangential speech A communication disorder in which the train of thought of the speaker wanders and shows a lack of focus, never returning to the initial topic of the conversation. It is less severe than logorrhea and may be associated with the middle stage in dementia. It is, however, more severe than circumstantial speech in which the speaker wanders, but eventually returns to the topic.

Tarasoff The lawsuit (Tarasoff v. Regents of the University of California) in which the Supreme Court of California held that mental health professionals have a duty to protect individuals who are being threatened with bodily harm by a patient. The original 1974 decision mandated warning the threatened individual, but a 1976 rehearing of the case by the California Supreme Court called for a "duty to protect" the intended victim. The professional may discharge the duty in several ways, including notifying police, warning the intended victim, and/or taking other reasonable steps to protect the threatened individual.

Veiled threats Coded statements in which no explicit intentions are articulated. This gives the utterer grounds for claiming that there was no legally actionable threat of harm. Veiled threats are similar to indirect ones when the exact consequences to the victim are ambiguous.

About the Author

Thomas Moll is a registered nurse who has a certification in psychiatric and mental health nursing from the Canadian Nurses Association and a board certification from the American Nurses Association. He is also holds certification from the National Commission on Correctional Health Care.

He currently works for the California Department of Corrections and Rehabilitation as a nurse consultant.

www.ingramcontent.com/pod-product-compliance
Lightning Source LLC
Chambersburg PA
CBHW052338220526
45472CB00001B/484